CHRONIC CONDITIONS AND THE MALE LIBIDO

Enduring Intimacy and Empowering Men To Confront Sexual Challenges Amidst Diabetes, Heart Diseases, Arthritis, And Chronic Pain.

Dr Wilson Nova

Table Of Contents

INTRODUCTION

CHAPTER 1

NAVIGATING THE CROSSROADS OF CHRONIC HEALTH AND SEXUAL WELLNESS

DISPELLING MYTHS AND CONFRONTING STIGMAS

CHAPTER 2

DIABETES AND LIBIDO: Understanding the Link and Reclaiming Intimacy

MANAGING BLOOD SUGAR LEVEL FOR OPTIMAL SEXUAL HEALTH

LIFESTYLE MODIFICATIONS FOR ENHANCING SEXUAL WELLNESS WITH DIABETES

CHAPTER THREE

HEART DISEASE AND YOUR SEX LIFE: Navigating Challenges and Restoring Passion

CHAPTER 4

ARTHRITIS AND SEXUAL HEALTH: Managing Symptoms and Maintaining Intimacy

CHAPTER 5

CHRONIC PAIN AND SEXUAL SATISFACTION: Strategies for Enhancing Pleasure and Connection

CHAPTER 6

SEXUAL WELLNESS IN MEN WITH MULTIPLE CHRONIC CONDITIONS:

CHAPTER 7

    EMBRACING WHOLENESS: A Path to Renewed Intimacy and Sexual Fulfillment.

CONCLUSION

    Empowering Men to Take Charge of Their Sexual Health

INTRODUCTION

In the realm of human health, sexual wellness is a fundamental aspect of overall well-being, encompassing physical, emotional, and psychological dimensions.

For men, a healthy libido, the natural desire for sexual intimacy, plays a crucial role in maintaining fulfilling relationships, experiencing pleasure, and fostering a sense of self-confidence. However, for many men living with chronic conditions, the path to sexual fulfilment can be challenging, often shrouded in misconceptions, stigma, and a lack of adequate support.

This book, "Chronic Conditions and the Male Libido," delves into the intricate interplay between chronic health issues and male sexual function, illuminating the often overlooked impact of these conditions on a man's intimate life. It aims to empower men with chronic conditions to reclaim their sexual wellness by providing comprehensive information, dispelling common myths, and offering practical strategies for managing sexual health challenges.

The Spectrum of Chronic Conditions and Their Impact on Libido

Chronic conditions, ranging from arthritis and diabetes to heart disease and chronic pain, can exert a significant influence on a man's libido. These conditions, often characterised by persistent pain, fatigue, and medication side effects, can disrupt the physical and psychological aspects of sexual desire, leading to feelings of frustration, inadequacy, and disconnection in relationships.

With this knowledge and guidance, you can reclaim your sexual wellness, maintain fulfilling relationships, and enhance your overall quality of life.

CHAPTER 1

NAVIGATING THE CROSSROADS OF CHRONIC HEALTH AND SEXUAL WELLNESS

Understanding the Intersection of Chronic Conditions and Male Libido

The intersection of chronic conditions and male libido is complex. Conditions like diabetes, cardiovascular issues, and obesity can impact hormonal balance and blood flow, affecting libido. Medications for chronic conditions may also have side effects. Lifestyle factors such as stress and lack of exercise play a role. It's crucial to address both the underlying health issues and consider holistic approaches to support male sexual health. Consulting with a healthcare professional is advisable for personalised guidance.

Chronic conditions can affect male libido through various mechanisms. Diabetes, for example, may lead to nerve damage and vascular issues, impacting blood flow to the genital area. Cardiovascular problems can also contribute to erectile dysfunction by compromising blood vessel function.

Hormonal imbalances, often associated with conditions like obesity or hypogonadism, can further influence libido. Testosterone, a key hormone for sexual function, may be reduced in such cases. Additionally, medications commonly prescribed for chronic conditions can have side effects on sexual health.

Beyond physiological factors, the psychological impact of chronic conditions can't be overlooked. Stress, anxiety, and depression, often associated with chronic illnesses, can contribute to a decline in libido.

Addressing these issues involves a comprehensive approach. Managing the chronic condition through medication and lifestyle changes is essential. Lifestyle modifications such as regular exercise, a balanced diet, and stress reduction techniques can positively impact both the chronic condition and libido.

Open communication with healthcare providers is crucial. They can offer tailored advice, potentially adjusting medications or recommending therapies to address specific aspects affecting libido. Overall, a holistic approach that considers both physical and mental well-being is key to managing the intersection of chronic conditions and male libido.

DISPELLING MYTHS AND CONFRONTING STIGMAS

Chronic health conditions and sexual dysfunction are often shrouded in myths and misconceptions, which can lead to unnecessary anxiety, embarrassment, and isolation. Addressing these myths and confronting the stigma associated with sexual challenges is crucial for men to seek help and reclaim their sexual wellness.

Myth 1: Erectile dysfunction is an inevitable part of aging.

Fact: While erectile dysfunction is more common among older men, it is not an inevitable consequence of aging. Many men with chronic health conditions can maintain a healthy sex life with proper management and treatment.

Myth 2: Only men with certain chronic conditions experience sexual problems.

Fact: Any chronic condition can potentially affect sexual function. The specific impact varies depending on the condition and its severity.

Myth 3: Sexual dysfunction is a sign of weakness or lack of masculinity.

Fact: Sexual dysfunction is a common symptom of many chronic health conditions and is not a reflection of a man's masculinity. Seeking help for sexual concerns is a sign of strength and commitment to one's overall health.

Myth 4: Talking about sexual problems is embarrassing and taboo.

Fact: Open communication about sexual concerns is essential for men to receive the support and treatment they need. Healthcare providers are trained to address sexual health issues and can provide a safe and comfortable environment for men to discuss their concerns.

Myth 5: There's nothing that can be done to improve sexual function with chronic health conditions.

Fact: With proper management and treatment, many men with chronic health conditions can enjoy a fulfilling sex life. Lifestyle changes, medication adjustments, and therapy can all contribute to improved sexual function.

Confronting Stigma

The stigma surrounding sexual dysfunction can prevent men from seeking help, leading to feelings of shame, isolation, and depression. This stigma can also contribute to delayed diagnosis and treatment, potentially worsening sexual problems.

Here are some ways to confront the stigma associated with sexual dysfunction:

- Educate yourself and others about chronic health conditions and their impact on sexual health.

- Talk openly and honestly about sexual concerns with your partner, healthcare providers, and friends or family members.

- Challenge negative stereotypes about sexual dysfunction and masculinity.

- Advocate for policies and programs that promote sexual health awareness and support for men with chronic health conditions.

By dispelling myths and confronting stigmas, we can create a more supportive and understanding environment for men to address their sexual health concerns and reclaim their sexual well-being.

Embracing a Holistic Approach to Sexual Health

Sexual health is an integral part of overall well-being, encompassing physical, psychological, and emotional aspects. A holistic approach to sexual health considers all these interconnected dimensions to promote a fulfilling and satisfying sex life.

Physical Aspects

Maintaining a healthy lifestyle: Engaging in regular physical activity, adopting a balanced diet, and getting adequate sleep contribute to overall physical health, which indirectly enhances sexual function.

Managing chronic conditions: Effectively managing chronic health conditions, such as diabetes, heart disease, or arthritis, can minimize their impact on sexual function and allow for a more fulfilling sex life.

Seeking medical guidance: Consulting with healthcare providers for regular checkups and addressing any sexual concerns promptly can help identify and address underlying

physical issues that may affect
sexual health.

Psychological Aspects

**Addressing stress and
anxiety:** Stress and anxiety can
significantly impact libido,
arousal, and sexual performance.
Practicing stress management
techniques, such as mindfulness
meditation or yoga, can help
reduce stress and promote
relaxation.

**Building self-esteem and
body image:** Positive
self-perception and body
acceptance can enhance sexual

confidence and contribute to a more fulfilling sex life. Challenging negative self-talk and practicing body positivity exercises can improve self-image.

Communicating openly and honestly: Open and honest communication with partners about sexual desires, preferences, and concerns can strengthen intimacy, reduce anxiety, and foster a more satisfying sex life.

Seeking professional support: If psychological factors, such as depression, anxiety, or past traumas, are affecting sexual health, seeking professional counseling or therapy can address these underlying issues.

Emotional Aspects

Nurturing emotional intimacy: Emotional intimacy, characterized by deep connection, trust, and mutual affection, forms the foundation for a fulfilling and passionate sex life. Spending quality time together, sharing feelings, and expressing appreciation can deepen emotional intimacy.

Cultivating a growth mindset: Approaching sexual challenges with a growth mindset, believing that abilities can be improved through effort and learning, can lead to a more positive and resilient attitude towards sexual health.

Embracing sensuality and pleasure: Focusing on sensuality and pleasure, rather than solely on performance, can enhance sexual satisfaction and reduce performance anxiety. Practicing mindfulness exercises and exploring different forms of touch and stimulation can increase sensuality.

Seeking support from partners and healthcare

providers: Open communication with partners about sexual concerns and seeking support from healthcare providers can help address emotional factors affecting sexual health.

A holistic approach to sexual health recognizes that sexual well-being is not solely determined by physical factors but is influenced by a complex interplay of physical, psychological, and emotional aspects. By addressing each of these dimensions, men with chronic health conditions can reclaim their sexual wellness and experience a fulfilling and satisfying sex life.

CHAPTER 2

DIABETES AND LIBIDO: Understanding the Link and Reclaiming Intimacy

Diabetes, a chronic metabolic disorder characterized by elevated blood sugar levels, can have a profound impact on a person's overall health and well-being, including their sexual function and libido. While the exact mechanisms are still being studied, research suggests that diabetes can affect libido in both men and women through various physiological and psychological pathways.

Physiological Effects of Diabetes on Libido

Nerve Damage: Diabetes can damage nerves throughout the body, including those involved in sexual arousal and function. This nerve damage can lead to erectile dysfunction (ED) in men and decreased vaginal lubrication in women.

Hormonal Imbalances: Diabetes can disrupt the delicate balance of hormones that regulate sexual function. For instance, high blood sugar levels can interfere with testosterone production in men, while low estrogen levels can contribute to decreased libido in women.

Blood Vessel Damage: Diabetes can damage blood vessels, reducing blood flow to the genitals. This impaired blood flow can make it difficult for men to achieve and maintain an erection and can also affect sexual sensation in both men and women.

Psychological Effects of Diabetes on Libido

Stress and Anxiety: The daily management of diabetes can be a significant source of stress and anxiety, which can negatively impact sexual desire.

Body Image Issues: Diabetes can lead to changes in body image and self-esteem, which can contribute to feelings of inadequacy and affect libido.

Relationship Strain: Diabetes can strain relationships, leading to communication problems and reduced intimacy, which can further impact libido.

Strategies for Reclaiming Intimacy

Despite the challenges posed by diabetes, there are effective strategies that men and women with diabetes can employ to reclaim their sexual health and intimacy.

Managing Blood Sugar Levels: Maintaining good blood sugar control is crucial for preventing or delaying nerve damage, hormonal imbalances, and blood vessel damage, all of which can contribute to sexual dysfunction.

Communicating with Healthcare Providers: Open and honest communication with healthcare providers about sexual concerns is essential for identifying underlying causes and developing a personalized treatment plan.

Adopting a Healthy Lifestyle: Engaging in regular exercise, eating a balanced diet, and getting adequate sleep can improve overall health and well-being, indirectly benefiting sexual function.

Stress Management Techniques: Practicing stress

management techniques, such as yoga, meditation, or deep breathing exercises, can help reduce stress and anxiety, which can improve libido.

Seeking Professional Support: If diabetes-related sexual concerns persist despite implementing these strategies, seeking professional support from a therapist or counselor can be beneficial.

Diabetes can affect libido, but it does not have to determine one's sexual health. By understanding the link between diabetes and libido, adopting healthy lifestyle habits, communicating openly with healthcare providers, and seeking professional support when needed, individuals with diabetes can reclaim their sexual wellness and maintain fulfilling and intimate relationships.

MANAGING BLOOD SUGAR LEVEL FOR OPTIMAL SEXUAL HEALTH

Diabetes, a chronic condition characterized by elevated blood sugar levels, can have a significant impact on a person's overall health and well-being, including their sexual function and libido. However, by maintaining good blood sugar control, individuals with diabetes can significantly improve their sexual health and enjoy a fulfilling intimate life.

The Impact of Blood Sugar Levels on Sexual Health

High blood sugar levels can damage nerves, blood vessels, and hormones throughout the body, all of which play a crucial role in sexual function. In men, nerve damage can lead to erectile dysfunction (ED), while hormonal imbalances can decrease testosterone levels and contribute to ED. In women, nerve damage can affect vaginal lubrication, and hormonal imbalances can reduce sexual desire and arousal.

Strategies for Managing Blood Sugar Levels

Effectively managing blood sugar levels is essential for preventing or delaying the complications of diabetes, including sexual dysfunction. Here are some key strategies for managing blood sugar levels:

1. Adherence to Medication: Taking prescribed medications as directed by healthcare providers is crucial for maintaining blood sugar control.

2. Regular Blood Sugar Monitoring: Regular self-monitoring of blood sugar levels allows individuals to track their progress and identify patterns that may require adjustments to their treatment plan.

3. Healthy Eating: A balanced diet rich in fruits, vegetables, whole grains, and lean protein helps regulate blood sugar levels and promotes overall health.

4. Regular Exercise: Engaging in regular physical activity, such as brisk walking, swimming, or cycling, improves insulin sensitivity and helps maintain blood sugar control.

5. Weight Management: Maintaining a healthy weight can significantly reduce the risk of diabetes complications, including sexual dysfunction.

Additional Tips for Optimal Sexual Health

- Communicate with Healthcare Providers: Open communication with healthcare providers about sexual concerns is essential for identifying underlying causes and developing a personalized treatment plan.

- Manage Stress: Stress can negatively impact blood sugar control and sexual function. Practicing stress management techniques, such as yoga, meditation, or deep breathing exercises, can be beneficial.

- Address Underlying Conditions: If other health conditions, such as high blood pressure or high cholesterol, are contributing to sexual dysfunction, managing these conditions is crucial.

- Seek Professional Support: If diabetes-related sexual concerns persist, seeking professional support from a therapist or counselor can be helpful.

Maintaining good blood sugar control is a cornerstone of managing diabetes and preventing its complications. By adhering to medication, monitoring blood sugar levels, adopting a healthy lifestyle, and seeking professional support when needed, individuals with diabetes can optimize their sexual health and enjoy a fulfilling intimate life. Remember, open communication with healthcare providers is essential for addressing sexual concerns and developing a personalized treatment plan.

LIFESTYLE MODIFICATIONS FOR ENHANCING SEXUAL WELLNESS WITH DIABETES

Dietary Changes:

- Prioritize Fruits, Vegetables, and Whole Grains: These nutrient-rich foods provide essential vitamins, minerals, and fiber, supporting overall health and sexual function.

- Choose Lean Protein Sources: Opt for lean meats, fish, poultry, and plant-based protein sources to maintain a healthy weight and support blood sugar control.

- Limit Saturated and Trans Fats: Reduce intake of saturated and trans fats, found in processed foods and red meats, as they can contribute to blood vessel damage and hinder sexual function.

- Moderate Sugar Intake: Minimize consumption of

added sugars, which can spike blood sugar levels and exacerbate diabetic complications.

Exercise and Physical Activity:

Engage in Regular Exercise: Aim for at least 150 minutes of moderate-intensity aerobic exercise per week, such as brisk walking, swimming, or cycling.

Incorporate Strength Training: Include strength training exercises at least twice a week to build muscle mass, which improves insulin sensitivity and overall health.

Find Enjoyable Activities: Choose physical activities you enjoy to make exercise a sustainable part of your lifestyle.

Stress Management:

- Practice Relaxation Techniques: Incorporate stress-management techniques, such as yoga, meditation, or deep breathing exercises, into your daily routine.

- Maintain a Healthy Sleep Schedule: Aim for 7-8 hours of quality sleep each night to allow your body to rest and repair, promoting overall well-being.

- Engage in Supportive Relationships: Nurture strong connections with loved ones to provide emotional support and reduce stress levels.

Communication and Intimacy:

Communicate Openly with Your Partner: Discuss sexual concerns openly and honestly with your partner to address any issues and foster intimacy.

Seek Professional Help: If communication challenges persist, consider seeking professional counseling to improve communication and strengthen your relationship.

Prioritize Quality Time Together: Schedule regular time for non-sexual activities with your partner to maintain emotional intimacy and connection.

Additional Considerations:

Monitor Blood Sugar Levels Regularly: Regularly check your blood sugar levels to track your progress and identify patterns that may require adjustments to your treatment plan.

Manage Other Health Conditions: Effectively manage other health conditions, such as high blood pressure or high cholesterol, as these can contribute to sexual dysfunction.

Avoid Smoking: Quitting smoking can significantly improve blood flow, reduce the risk of nerve damage, and enhance overall health, including sexual function.

Moderate Alcohol Consumption: Excessive alcohol intake can interfere with blood sugar control and sexual function. Limit alcohol consumption or avoid it altogether.

Remember, these lifestyle modifications should be tailored to your individual needs and preferences. Consult your healthcare provider to develop a personalized plan that suits your specific situation and goals.

CHAPTER THREE

HEART DISEASE AND YOUR SEX LIFE: Navigating Challenges and Restoring Passion

Cardiovascular health, encompassing the health of the heart and blood vessels, plays a crucial role in maintaining overall well-being, including sexual health. A strong cardiovascular system ensures adequate blood flow to various organs, including the genitals, which is essential for sexual function. Conversely, cardiovascular diseases, such as coronary artery disease (CAD) and peripheral artery disease (PAD), can significantly impact male libido and sexual performance.

Impact of Cardiovascular Diseases on Male Libido

1. Reduced Blood Flow: Cardiovascular diseases can damage blood vessels, leading to impaired blood flow to the genitals. This impaired blood flow can make it difficult for men to achieve and maintain an erection, a condition known as erectile dysfunction (ED).

2. Hormonal Imbalances: Certain medications used to treat cardiovascular diseases, such as beta-blockers and diuretics, can have side effects that affect sexual function. For instance, beta-blockers can reduce testosterone levels, while diuretics can decrease libido.

3. Psychological Factors: Cardiovascular diseases can cause stress, anxiety, and depression, which can negatively impact libido and sexual desire.

Strategies for Enhancing Cardiovascular Health and Improving Male Libido

1. Lifestyle Modifications: Adopting a healthy lifestyle, including a balanced diet, regular exercise, and adequate sleep, can significantly improve cardiovascular health and reduce the risk of ED.

2. Managing Chronic Conditions: Effectively managing chronic conditions, such as diabetes and high blood pressure, can minimize their impact on cardiovascular health and sexual function.

3. Open Communication with Healthcare Providers: Open and honest communication with healthcare providers about sexual concerns is essential for identifying underlying causes and developing a personalized treatment plan.

4. Stress Management Techniques: Practicing stress management techniques, such as yoga, meditation, or deep breathing exercises, can help reduce stress and anxiety, which can improve libido.

5. Seeking Professional Support: If cardiovascular-related sexual concerns persist despite implementing these strategies, seeking professional support from a therapist or counselor can be beneficial.

Maintaining a healthy cardiovascular system is crucial for overall well-being and sexual health in men. By adopting a healthy lifestyle, managing chronic conditions, and addressing sexual concerns with healthcare providers, men can effectively manage cardiovascular risk factors, improve blood flow, and reclaim their sexual function. Remember, open communication and seeking professional support when needed are key to optimizing sexual health and overall well-being.

Addressing Sexual Side Effects of Heart Disease Medications

Heart disease medications play a vital role in managing cardiovascular conditions and reducing the risk of complications. However, some medications used to treat heart disease can have side effects that affect sexual function, including decreased libido and erectile dysfunction (ED).

Common Medications with Sexual Side Effects

Beta-blockers: These medications, such as atenolol (Tenormin) and metoprolol (Lopressor), slow down the heart rate and reduce blood pressure. However, they can also block the release of nitric oxide, a substance essential for erectile function.

Diuretics: These medications, such as hydrochlorothiazide (HydroDIURIL) and furosemide (Lasix), help remove excess fluid from the body. However, they can also cause potassium loss, which can contribute to ED.

Antihypertensives: These medications, such as ACE

inhibitors and angiotensin II receptor blockers (ARBs), lower blood pressure. While generally well-tolerated, some may cause ED as a side effect.

Strategies for Managing Medication-Related Sexual Side Effects

1. Communicate with Your Healthcare Provider: Open and honest communication with your doctor is crucial for addressing sexual concerns related to medications. Discussing your symptoms and libido changes can help determine if your medications are contributing to the issue.

2. Explore Medication Adjustments: Your doctor may consider adjusting the dosage or timing of your medication to minimize side effects. In some cases, switching to a different medication with fewer sexual side effects may be an option.

3. Lifestyle Modifications: Adopting a healthy lifestyle, including regular exercise, a balanced diet, and adequate sleep, can improve overall health and potentially reduce the impact of medication side effects on libido.

4. Stress Management: Stress can exacerbate sexual dysfunction. Practicing stress management techniques, such as yoga, meditation, or deep breathing exercises, can help reduce stress and improve libido.

5. Professional Support: If sexual concerns persist despite implementing these strategies, seeking professional support from a therapist or counselor can be beneficial. They can provide counseling and address underlying psychological factors that may affect libido.

Heart disease medications can play a crucial role in managing cardiovascular health, but it's important to be aware of potential side effects on sexual function. Open communication with your healthcare provider is essential for identifying and addressing these side effects. By working with your doctor, making lifestyle changes, and seeking professional support when needed, men can effectively manage medication side effects and maintain a fulfilling sexual life. Remember, treating the underlying heart condition is paramount for long-term health and well-being.

Embracing a Heart-Healthy Lifestyle for Enhanced Sexual Function

Maintaining a healthy heart is not just about preventing cardiovascular diseases; it's also about promoting overall well-being, including sexual health. A heart-healthy lifestyle, characterized by nutritious eating habits, regular exercise, and adequate rest, can significantly improve sexual function and enhance intimacy.

The Link Between Heart Health and Sexual Function

The heart plays a crucial role in sexual function by ensuring adequate blood flow to the genitals. This blood flow is essential for achieving and maintaining an erection in men and for vaginal lubrication in women. When heart health is compromised, blood flow can be impaired, leading to sexual dysfunction.

Heart-Healthy Habits for Enhanced Sexual Function

1. Adopt a Balanced Diet: Prioritize fruits, vegetables, whole grains, and lean protein sources to provide essential nutrients for overall health and sexual function. Limit processed foods, saturated and trans fats, and added sugars, as they can contribute to cardiovascular diseases and sexual dysfunction.

2. Engage in Regular Exercise: Aim for at least 150 minutes of moderate-intensity aerobic exercise per week, such as brisk walking, swimming, or cycling. Regular physical activity improves blood flow, reduces stress, and enhances overall well-being, all of which can benefit sexual function.

3. Maintain a Healthy Weight: Excess weight can contribute to cardiovascular diseases, which can indirectly affect sexual function. Aim for a healthy weight range and avoid unhealthy weight loss methods.

4. Quit Smoking: Smoking damages blood vessels and reduces blood flow, increasing the risk of cardiovascular diseases and erectile dysfunction. Quitting smoking is a significant step towards improving both heart health and sexual function.

5. Moderate Alcohol Consumption: Excessive alcohol

intake can interfere with blood sugar control, blood pressure, and sexual function. Limit alcohol consumption or avoid it altogether for optimal sexual health.

6. Manage Stress Effectively: Chronic stress can negatively impact blood flow, reduce testosterone levels, and contribute to sexual dysfunction. Practice stress management techniques, such as yoga, meditation, or deep breathing exercises, to promote relaxation and improve sexual function.

7. Adequate Sleep: Aim for 7-8 hours of quality sleep each night to allow your body to rest and repair, promoting overall well-being and sexual function.

8. Communicate with Your Healthcare Provider: Open communication with your doctor about sexual concerns is essential for identifying underlying causes and developing a personalized treatment plan.

Embracing a heart-healthy lifestyle is a holistic approach to maintaining overall health and enhancing sexual function. By adopting a balanced diet, engaging in regular exercise, managing stress effectively, and communicating openly with your healthcare provider, you can promote a healthy cardiovascular system, improve blood flow, and reclaim a fulfilling sexual life. Remember, a heart-healthy lifestyle is not just about preventing future complications; it's about enjoying a vibrant and fulfilling present.

CHAPTER 4

ARTHRITIS AND SEXUAL HEALTH: Managing Symptoms and Maintaining Intimacy

Arthritis, a condition characterized by inflammation and pain in the joints, can significantly impact various aspects of life, including sexual function. While the exact mechanisms are still being studied, research suggests that arthritis can affect male sexual function through physical, psychological, and emotional pathways.

Physical Effects of Arthritis on Male Sexual Function

Pain and Stiffness: Arthritis-related pain and stiffness in the joints can make it difficult to find comfortable positions for sexual activity and can hinder arousal and orgasm.

Nerve Damage: Arthritis can damage nerves in the pelvic area, which can lead to erectile dysfunction (ED), characterized by the inability to achieve or maintain an erection.

Medications: Some medications used to treat arthritis, such as nonsteroidal anti-inflammatory drugs (NSAIDs), can have side effects that affect sexual function.

Psychological Effects of Arthritis on Male Sexual Function

Stress and Anxiety: The daily management of arthritis can be a source of stress and anxiety, which can negatively impact libido and sexual performance.

Body Image Issues: Arthritis can lead to changes in body image and self-esteem, which can contribute to feelings of inadequacy and affect libido.

Relationship Strain: Arthritis-related pain and discomfort can strain relationships, leading to communication problems and reduced intimacy, which can further impact libido.

Strategies for Managing Arthritis and Improving Sexual Health

Effective Pain Management: Working with healthcare providers to manage arthritis pain effectively can make sexual activity more comfortable and improve overall well-being.

Open Communication with Partners: Open and honest communication with partners about sexual concerns is essential for understanding each other's needs and finding ways to maintain intimacy.

Exploring Alternative Positions: Experimenting with different sexual positions that minimize strain on affected joints can make sexual activity more enjoyable and comfortable.

Seeking Professional Support: If sexual concerns persist despite implementing these strategies, seeking professional support from a therapist or counselor can be beneficial. They can provide counseling and address underlying psychological factors that may affect libido.

Arthritis can pose challenges to male sexual function, but it does not have to determine one's sexual health. By understanding the link between arthritis and sexual function, adopting proactive pain management strategies, communicating openly with partners, and seeking professional support when needed, men with arthritis can reclaim their sexual wellness and maintain fulfilling intimate relationships.

Coping with Pain and Inflammation for Sexual Wellness

Pain and inflammation can significantly impact various aspects of life, including sexual function. Chronic pain conditions like arthritis, inflammatory bowel disease, and fibromyalgia can make it difficult to engage in sexual activity due to discomfort, fatigue, and emotional distress.

However, there are strategies that individuals with pain and inflammation can employ to manage their symptoms and maintain a fulfilling sexual life.

Understanding the Impact of Pain and Inflammation

Pain and inflammation can affect sexual health in several ways:

Physical discomfort: Pain in the joints, muscles, or genitals can make it difficult to find comfortable positions for sexual activity.

Reduced libido: Pain and inflammation can contribute to fatigue, anxiety, and stress, which can negatively impact libido and sexual desire.

Medications: Some medications used to treat pain and inflammation can have side effects that affect sexual function, such as erectile dysfunction or decreased vaginal lubrication.

Strategies for Managing Pain and Inflammation

Effective pain management is crucial for improving sexual health and overall well-being.

Here are some strategies to consider:

Work with your healthcare providers: Collaborate with your doctor, physical therapist, and other healthcare professionals to develop a personalized pain management plan that addresses your specific needs and condition.

Explore pain management techniques: Consider incorporating non-pharmacological pain management techniques into your routine, such as yoga, meditation, acupuncture, or massage therapy.

Manage stress effectively: Chronic pain can contribute to stress, which can exacerbate pain and negatively impact sexual function. Practice stress management techniques, such as deep breathing exercises or mindfulness meditation, to reduce stress levels.

Communicate openly with your partner: Open and honest communication with your partner about your pain and sexual concerns is essential for understanding each other's needs and finding ways to maintain intimacy.

Seek professional support: If sexual concerns persist despite implementing these strategies, seeking professional support from a therapist or counselor can be beneficial. They can provide counseling and address underlying psychological factors that may affect libido.

Enhancing Sexual Wellness

In addition to managing pain, there are specific steps that individuals with pain and inflammation can take to enhance their sexual wellness:

Prioritize intimacy: Make time for non-sexual activities with your partner to nurture intimacy and emotional connection, which can contribute to a fulfilling sex life.

Explore alternative positions: Experiment with different sexual positions that minimize strain on affected joints or areas of pain.

Use lubricants: If vaginal dryness is an issue, consider using lubricants to enhance comfort and pleasure.

Be patient and understanding: Understand that sexual activity may need to be adapted to accommodate pain levels and energy limitations.

Remember, communication, understanding, and a willingness to experiment are key to maintaining a fulfilling sexual life despite pain and inflammation. With the right support and strategies, individuals can manage their symptoms and reclaim their sexual wellness.

Lifestyle Strategies for Enhancing Intimacy with Arthritis

Arthritis, a condition characterized by inflammation

and pain in the joints, can pose challenges to intimacy and sexual relationships. However, by adopting effective pain management strategies, prioritizing communication, and exploring alternative approaches to intimacy, individuals with arthritis can maintain fulfilling and meaningful connections with their partners.

Managing Pain and Inflammation for Intimacy

Effective Pain Management: Work with healthcare providers to develop a personalized pain management plan that addresses your specific needs and condition. This may include medication, physical therapy, and non-pharmacological techniques like yoga, meditation, or massage therapy.

Prioritize Sleep: Adequate sleep is crucial for both physical and emotional well-being. Aim for 7-8 hours of quality sleep each night to allow your body to rest and repair, reducing fatigue and improving overall well-being.

Maintain a Healthy Weight: Excess weight can put additional strain on affected joints, exacerbating pain and discomfort.

Aim for a healthy weight range to reduce joint stress and improve overall health.

Regular Exercise: Engaging in regular physical activity, such as low-impact exercises like swimming or walking, can strengthen muscles around affected joints, improve flexibility, and reduce pain.

Nurturing Connection and Intimacy

Open Communication: Open and honest communication with your partner about your pain, concerns, and needs is essential for fostering understanding and support.

Plan Intimate Moments: Schedule time for non-sexual activities with your partner to strengthen your bond and create opportunities for intimacy.

Express Affection: Non-sexual forms of affection, such as cuddling, holding hands, or giving compliments, can enhance emotional intimacy and strengthen your relationship.

Seek Professional Support: If communication challenges persist or emotional distress affects your relationship, consider seeking professional counseling to address underlying issues.

Exploring Alternative Approaches to Intimacy

Sensual Exploration: Focus on sensual experiences, such as massage, touch, and gentle caresses, to build arousal and intimacy without relying solely on intercourse.

Communication-Based Intimacy: Explore non-physical forms of intimacy, such as sharing fantasies, talking about your relationship, and expressing your feelings, to deepen your connection.

Experiment with Positions: Try different sexual positions that minimize strain on affected joints and find comfortable ways to be intimate.

Utilize Lubricants: If vaginal dryness is an issue, consider using lubricants to enhance comfort and pleasure.

Remember

Patience and Understanding: Sexual activity may need to be adapted to accommodate pain levels and energy limitations. Be patient with yourself and your partner, and focus on shared pleasure and connection.

Seek Support: Don't hesitate to seek support from healthcare providers, therapists, or support groups to address both physical and emotional challenges.

Embrace Flexibility: Be open to exploring different ways of expressing intimacy and find what works best for you and your partner.

By adopting effective pain management strategies,

prioritizing communication, and exploring alternative approaches to intimacy, individuals with arthritis can maintain fulfilling and meaningful connections with their partners, enhancing their overall well-being and quality of life.

CHAPTER 5

CHRONIC PAIN AND SEXUAL SATISFACTION: Strategies for Enhancing Pleasure and Connection

Navigating the Complexities of Chronic Pain and Male Libido

Chronic pain, a persistent and often debilitating condition, can significantly impact various aspects of life, including sexual health and libido. The intricate connection between chronic pain and male libido involves a complex interplay of physical, psychological, and emotional factors.

Physical Effects of Chronic Pain on Libido

Painful Sensations: The constant presence of pain can make it difficult to focus on sexual arousal and pleasure, hindering libido and sexual function.

Reduced Energy Levels: Chronic pain can lead to fatigue and exhaustion, making it challenging to engage in physical activities, including sexual intimacy.

Medications: Some medications used to manage chronic pain, such as opioids and antidepressants, can have side effects that negatively impact libido and sexual function.

Psychological Effects of Chronic Pain on Libido

Stress and Anxiety: The daily stress of managing chronic pain can contribute to anxiety and depression, which can further suppress libido and sexual desire.

Body Image Issues: Chronic pain can lead to changes in body image and self-esteem, affecting how individuals perceive their attractiveness and desirability, potentially impacting libido.

Relationship Strain: Chronic pain can strain relationships, leading to communication problems and reduced intimacy, which can further impact libido.

Strategies for Managing Chronic Pain and Improving Libido

Effective Pain Management: Working closely with healthcare providers to develop a personalized pain management plan that addresses specific pain levels and underlying conditions can significantly improve overall well-being and enhance libido.

Open Communication with Partners: Open and honest communication with partners about pain concerns and sexual needs is crucial for understanding each other's perspectives and finding ways to maintain intimacy.

Exploring Alternative Positions: Experimenting with different sexual positions that minimize strain on affected areas can make sexual activity more comfortable and enjoyable.

Prioritizing Intimacy: Nurturing non-sexual intimacy through shared activities, emotional connection, and expressing affection can strengthen the bond with your partner and enhance overall intimacy.

Seeking Professional Support: If chronic pain or sexual concerns persist despite implementing these strategies, seeking professional support from a therapist or counselor can be beneficial. They can address underlying psychological factors that may affect libido.

Chronic pain can pose challenges to male libido, but it does not have to define one's sexual health. By understanding the link between chronic pain and libido, adopting effective pain management strategies, communicating openly with partners, and seeking professional support when needed, men can reclaim their sexual wellness and maintain fulfilling intimate relationships. Remember, chronic pain is a complex condition, and addressing it requires a multifaceted approach that encompasses physical, psychological, and emotional well-being.

Addressing Pain Management for Improved Sexual Function

Pain, whether acute or chronic, can significantly impact various aspects of life, including sexual function and overall well-being. While pain can manifest in diverse forms, ranging from joint pain to neuropathic discomfort, it can disrupt the physical and emotional aspects of intimacy, hindering sexual desire and enjoyment. However, by adopting effective pain management strategies and fostering open communication, individuals can reclaim their sexual wellness and maintain fulfilling relationships.

The Interplay of Pain and Sexual Function

Pain can affect sexual function in several ways:

Physical Discomfort: Painful sensations can make it difficult to find comfortable positions for sexual activity, leading to discomfort and inhibiting arousal.

Reduced Libido: Chronic pain can contribute to fatigue, stress, and anxiety, which can negatively impact libido and sexual desire.

Medications: Some medications used to manage pain, such as certain antidepressants and opioids, can have side effects that affect sexual function, such as erectile dysfunction or decreased vaginal lubrication.

Strategies for Effective Pain Management

Effective pain management is crucial for improving sexual function and overall well-being.

Here are some strategies to consider:

Collaborative Pain Management Plan: Work with your healthcare providers to develop a personalized pain management plan that addresses your specific needs and condition. This may include medication, physical therapy, and non-pharmacological techniques like yoga, meditation, or massage therapy.

Prioritize Sleep: Adequate sleep is essential for both physical and emotional well-being, allowing your body to rest and repair, reducing fatigue and improving overall well-being.

Maintain a Healthy Weight: Excess weight can put additional strain on affected joints or areas of pain, exacerbating discomfort. Aim for a healthy weight range to reduce strain and improve overall health.

Regular Exercise: Engaging in regular physical activity, such as low-impact exercises like swimming or walking, can strengthen muscles around affected areas, improve flexibility, and reduce pain.

Nurturing Intimacy and Sexual Wellness

In addition to managing pain, there are specific steps that individuals can take to enhance their sexual wellness:

Open Communication: Open and honest communication with your partner about your pain, concerns, and needs is essential for fostering understanding and support.

Plan Intimate Moments: Schedule time for non-sexual activities with your partner to strengthen your bond and create opportunities for intimacy.

Express Affection: Non-sexual forms of affection, such as cuddling, holding hands, or giving compliments, can enhance emotional intimacy and strengthen your relationship.

Explore Alternative Approaches: Experiment with different sexual positions that minimize strain on affected areas and find comfortable ways to be intimate.

Utilization of Lubricants: If vaginal dryness is an issue, consider using lubricants to enhance comfort and pleasure.

Remember

Patience and Understanding: Sexual activity may need to be adapted to accommodate pain levels and energy limitations. Be patient with yourself and your partner, and focus on shared pleasure and connection.

Seek Support: Don't hesitate to seek support from healthcare providers, therapists, or support groups to address both physical and emotional challenges.

Embrace Flexibility: Be open to exploring different ways of expressing intimacy and find what works best for you and your partner.

By adopting effective pain management strategies, prioritizing communication, and exploring alternative approaches to intimacy, individuals can reclaim their sexual wellness and maintain fulfilling relationships, enhancing their overall quality of life

Fostering Emotional Connection and Intimacy Amidst Chronic Pain

Chronic pain can undoubtedly pose challenges to emotional connection and intimacy. The constant presence of pain can be emotionally draining, leading to fatigue, anxiety, and social withdrawal. However, it's important to remember that chronic pain doesn't have to define your relationships or hinder your ability to form meaningful connections. By prioritizing communication, practicing self-care, and seeking support when needed, you can maintain strong and fulfilling relationships despite the challenges of chronic pain.

Communication is Key

Open and honest communication with your partner is crucial for navigating the complexities of chronic pain and maintaining emotional intimacy. Share your concerns about how pain affects you physically and emotionally, and be open to hearing their perspective. Together, you can explore ways to adapt your relationship and intimacy to accommodate your pain levels and limitations.

Prioritize Self-Care

Taking care of yourself is essential for maintaining your emotional well-being and fostering healthy relationships. Engage in activities that bring you joy and relaxation, whether it's reading, listening to music, spending time in nature, or practicing mindfulness. Prioritize adequate sleep, a healthy diet, and regular physical activity, as these can all contribute to improved energy levels and emotional resilience.

Seek Support When Needed

Don't hesitate to seek support from healthcare providers, therapists, or support groups to address both physical and emotional challenges. Talking to professionals can provide valuable coping strategies, emotional support, and guidance for navigating the complexities of chronic pain and relationships.

Remember, you are not alone

Many people experience chronic pain and face similar challenges in their relationships. Connecting with others who understand your situation can provide a sense of community, validation, and valuable insights. Consider joining support groups or online forums to connect with others who share your experiences.

Embrace Flexibility

Chronic pain may require adapting your approach to intimacy and connection. Be open to exploring different ways of expressing affection and intimacy, such as non-sexual touch, shared activities, and meaningful conversations. Focus on fostering emotional closeness and shared experiences, rather than solely relying on physical intimacy.

Patience and Understanding

Managing chronic pain and maintaining relationships require patience and understanding from both partners. Be patient with yourself and your partner as you navigate the challenges together. Celebrate small victories and focus on shared moments of connection and joy.

By prioritizing communication, practicing self-care, seeking support, and embracing flexibility, you can nurture strong and fulfilling relationships amidst chronic pain. Remember, emotional connection and intimacy are essential aspects of human well-being, and they can

thrive even in the face of
challenges.

CHAPTER 6

SEXUAL WELLNESS IN MEN WITH MULTIPLE CHRONIC CONDITIONS:

Juggling multiple chronic conditions can pose significant challenges to overall health and well-being, including sexual function and intimacy. However, adopting a proactive approach to managing chronic conditions and prioritizing sexual health can significantly improve the quality of life for individuals living with multiple conditions.

Understanding the Impact of Multiple Chronic Conditions on Sexual Health

Multiple chronic conditions, such as diabetes, heart disease, arthritis, and chronic pain, can affect sexual health in several ways:

Physical discomfort: Pain, fatigue, and other physical symptoms can make it difficult to find comfortable positions for sexual activity and can hinder arousal and orgasm.

Reduced libido: Chronic conditions can contribute to

stress, anxiety, and depression, which can negatively impact libido and sexual desire.

Medications: Many medications used to manage chronic conditions can have side effects that affect sexual function, such as erectile dysfunction or decreased vaginal lubrication.

Strategies for Managing Multiple Chronic Conditions and Improving Sexual Health

1. Effective Pain Management: Work with healthcare providers to develop a personalized pain management plan that addresses your specific needs and conditions. This may include medication, physical therapy, and non-pharmacological techniques like yoga, meditation, or massage therapy.

2. Prioritize Sleep: Adequate sleep is essential for both physical and emotional well-being, allowing your body to rest and repair, reducing fatigue and improving overall well-being.

3. Maintain a Healthy Weight: Excess weight can exacerbate joint pain, fatigue, and other symptoms of chronic conditions. Aim for a healthy weight range to reduce strain and improve overall health.

4. Regular Exercise: Engaging in regular physical activity, even low-impact exercises like swimming or walking, can strengthen muscles, improve flexibility, and reduce pain.

5. Open Communication with Partners: Open and honest communication with partners about your pain, concerns, and needs is essential for fostering understanding and support.

6. Explore Alternative Positions: Experimenting with

different sexual positions that minimize strain on affected areas can make sexual activity more comfortable and enjoyable.

7. Utilize Lubricants: If vaginal dryness is an issue, consider using lubricants to enhance comfort and pleasure.

8. Seek Professional Support: If sexual concerns persist despite implementing these strategies, seeking professional support from a therapist or counselor can be beneficial. They can address underlying psychological factors that may affect libido and provide guidance for improving sexual communication and intimacy.

Additional Tips for Enhancing Sexual Wellness

Prioritize Intimacy: Nurture non-sexual intimacy through shared activities, emotional connection, and expressing affection to strengthen your bond with your partner.

Communicate with Healthcare Providers: Discuss sexual concerns openly and honestly with your healthcare providers. They can provide personalized advice and help manage medication side effects.

Embrace Flexibility: Be open to exploring different ways of expressing intimacy and find what works best for you and your partner.

Seek Support Groups: Consider joining support groups or online forums to connect with others who share your experiences and gain valuable insights.

Remember, managing multiple chronic conditions and maintaining sexual health requires a holistic approach that encompasses physical, psychological, and emotional well-being. By adopting effective pain management strategies, prioritizing communication, practicing self-care, and seeking professional support when needed, individuals can reclaim their sexual wellness and maintain fulfilling relationships.

The Importance of Communication and Open Dialogue

Communication and open dialogue are fundamental pillars of any successful relationship, whether personal, professional, or otherwise. They enable individuals to connect, share ideas, resolve conflicts, and build strong bonds. Effective communication fosters understanding, empathy, and trust, creating a foundation for mutually beneficial interactions.

Key Benefits of Communication and Open Dialogue

1. Strengthened Relationships: Open communication fosters deeper connections and understanding between individuals, nurturing trust and intimacy. It allows for the sharing of thoughts, feelings, and concerns, promoting empathy and a sense of being heard.

2. Enhanced Problem-Solving: Effective communication facilitates collaborative problem-solving, enabling individuals to address issues constructively and find mutually agreeable solutions. Open dialogue encourages different perspectives and approaches, leading to more informed decisions.

3. Reduced Conflict and Misunderstandings: Open communication helps prevent misunderstandings and conflicts by clarifying intentions, addressing concerns promptly, and resolving disagreements respectfully. It allows individuals to express their needs and expectations clearly, minimizing the likelihood of misinterpretations.

4. Improved Personal Growth: Open dialogue encourages individuals to share their experiences, seek feedback, and learn from others. It fosters a supportive environment for personal growth and development, enabling individuals to gain new insights and perspectives.

5. Effective Teamwork and Collaboration: In professional settings, open communication and dialogue are essential for successful teamwork and collaboration. They promote information sharing, coordination of efforts, and alignment of goals, leading to better outcomes.

Strategies for Enhancing Communication and Open Dialogue

1. Active Listening: Practice active listening by giving undivided attention to the speaker, maintaining eye contact, and avoiding interrupting. Show empathy and understanding by reflecting back what you have heard and asking clarifying questions.

2. Clarity and Directness: Communicate clearly and directly, expressing your thoughts and feelings in a concise and understandable manner. Avoid ambiguity and vagueness, and be mindful of your tone and body language.

3. Respectful Disagreements: Recognize that differences in opinions are natural, and approach disagreements with respect and understanding. Listen to opposing viewpoints, acknowledge their validity, and seek common ground for compromise.

4. Non-Verbal Communication: Be aware of the impact of non-verbal cues, such as facial expressions, gestures, and posture. Maintain a positive and open body language to convey your willingness to engage in an open dialogue.

5. Seek Professional Support: If communication challenges persist or hinder relationships, consider seeking professional support from a therapist or counselor. They can provide guidance on effective communication techniques and conflict resolution strategies.

Communication and open dialogue are essential skills that empower individuals to connect, collaborate, and thrive in various aspects of life. By prioritizing open communication, actively listening, and approaching interactions with respect and empathy, individuals can build strong relationships, resolve conflicts constructively, and achieve personal and collective success.

CHAPTER 7

EMBRACING WHOLENESS: A Path to Renewed Intimacy and Sexual Fulfillment.

Sexual wellness is often portrayed as a state of physical and emotional well-being that allows individuals to have fulfilling and enjoyable sexual experiences. However, for many people living with chronic health challenges, traditional definitions of sexual wellness can feel restrictive and unattainable. Chronic conditions, such as pain, fatigue, and medication side effects, can significantly impact sexual function and intimacy, leading to feelings of frustration, inadequacy, and disconnection.

Reframing Sexual Wellness

Rather than adhering to rigid standards of sexual performance or pleasure, it is crucial to redefine sexual wellness in a way that is inclusive and empowering for individuals facing chronic health challenges. Sexual wellness should not be solely defined by the ability to engage in intercourse or achieve orgasm; instead, it should encompass a broader spectrum of experiences that promote intimacy, connection, and self-expression.

Prioritizing Self-Compassion and Understanding

Chronic health conditions can take a toll on self-esteem and body image, making it challenging to feel comfortable and confident in one's own skin. Practicing self-compassion and self-acceptance is essential for reclaiming sexual wellness. Acknowledge your limitations and challenges without self-judgment, and focus on aspects of your body and yourself that you appreciate.

Open Communication and Partnership

Open and honest communication with your partner is crucial for navigating the complexities of chronic health conditions and sexual wellness. Discuss your concerns, fears, and preferences openly, and work together to find ways to adapt and maintain intimacy.

Exploring Alternative Expressions of Intimacy

Sexual wellness encompasses a wide range of expressions beyond intercourse. Explore non-sexual forms of intimacy, such as cuddling, massage, shared activities, and emotional connection. Focus on building a sense of closeness and shared pleasure rather than solely relying on physical intimacy.

Exploring Alternative Positions and Lubricants

Painful sensations during sexual activity can be a significant barrier to sexual wellness. Experiment with different sexual positions that minimize strain on affected areas and explore the use of lubricants to enhance comfort and pleasure.

Seeking Professional Support

If sexual concerns persist despite implementing these strategies, seeking professional support from a therapist or counselor can be beneficial. They can provide guidance on effective communication techniques, address underlying psychological factors that may affect libido, and help you develop personalized strategies for enhancing sexual wellness.

Remember, sexual wellness is a journey, not a destination.It is about finding ways to express intimacy, pleasure, and connection in a way that aligns with your unique needs and limitations. By embracing self-compassion, communicating openly with your partner, and exploring alternative approaches to intimacy, you can reclaim your sexual wellness and maintain fulfilling relationships, even in the face of chronic health challenges.

Cultivating Self-Compassion and Body Acceptance

In a world that constantly bombards us with unrealistic beauty standards and messages of perfection, it's easy to fall into the trap of self-criticism and body dissatisfaction. However, cultivating self-compassion and body acceptance is essential for our emotional and mental well-being, allowing us to embrace our bodies and ourselves just as we are.

Understanding Self-Compassion and Body Acceptance

Self-compassion is the practice of treating oneself with kindness, understanding, and acceptance, especially when facing imperfections or setbacks. It involves recognizing that everyone experiences challenges and flaws, and that we are worthy of love and respect, regardless of our appearance or achievements.

Body acceptance, on the other hand, is the process of coming to terms with our physical appearance and appreciating our bodies for their unique beauty and functionality. It's about moving beyond societal expectations and embracing our individual bodies, with all their imperfections and quirks.

The Benefits of Self-Compassion and Body Acceptance

Cultivating self-compassion and body acceptance has numerous benefits for our overall well-being. These include:

Reduced Self-Criticism and Negative Thoughts: Self-compassion helps us silence our inner critic and view ourselves with more kindness and understanding, leading to a reduction in negative self-talk and improved self-esteem.

Enhanced Emotional Resilience: Self-compassion allows us to navigate challenges and setbacks with greater resilience, enabling us to bounce back from disappointments and setbacks more effectively.

Improved Mental Health: Self-compassion and body acceptance are linked to reduced symptoms of depression, anxiety, and eating disorders, promoting a more positive and balanced mental state.

Stronger Relationships: Self-compassion fosters healthier and more fulfilling relationships, as we are better able to extend kindness and understanding to others, including our partners and friends.

Strategies for Cultivating Self-Compassion and Body Acceptance

1. Practice Self-Awareness: Pay attention to your thoughts and feelings towards yourself, particularly when you engage in self-criticism. Acknowledge these thoughts without judgment, and remind yourself that everyone has flaws and imperfections.

2. Challenge Negative Self-Talk: Replace negative self-talk with more positive and compassionate affirmations. Instead of focusing on your flaws, remind yourself of your strengths, qualities, and accomplishments.

3. Practice Mindfulness: Engage in mindfulness exercises, such as meditation or yoga, to cultivate present-moment awareness and reduce judgmental thoughts.

4. Engage in Self-Care: Prioritize activities that nurture your body and mind, such as exercise, healthy eating, and getting enough sleep. Self-care demonstrates your commitment to your well-being.

5. Surround Yourself with Positivity: Limit your exposure to negative media messages and surround yourself with supportive people who encourage self-acceptance and body positivity.

6. Seek Professional Support: If you struggle with persistent negative self-talk or low self-esteem, consider seeking professional help from a therapist or counselor. They can provide guidance and support in developing self-compassion and body acceptance strategies.

Remember, cultivating self-compassion and body acceptance is a journey, not a destination. It takes time, effort, and self-awareness to break free from negative self-perceptions and embrace your body with kindness and acceptance. Be patient with yourself, celebrate your progress, and focus on the positive aspects of yourself and your body. With consistent effort, you can develop a deeper sense of self-love and body appreciation, leading to a more fulfilling and joyful life.

CONCLUSION

Empowering Men to Take Charge of Their Sexual Health

Sexual health is an integral part of overall well-being, encompassing physical, emotional, and mental aspects of a man's intimate life. However, many men hesitate to seek help or prioritize their sexual health, leading to preventable issues and impacting their quality of life. Empowering men to take charge of their sexual health is crucial for fostering open communication, promoting early intervention, and ensuring men receive the support they need to maintain a fulfilling and healthy sex life.

Breaking Down Barriers to Men's Sexual Health

Several factors contribute to men's reluctance to address sexual health concerns, including:

Stigma and Embarrassment: Societal expectations and stereotypes often lead men to feel ashamed or embarrassed about discussing sexual issues, hindering open communication and seeking help.

Lack of Awareness: Many men lack adequate knowledge about sexual health and the importance of regular checkups, making them less likely to prioritize preventive measures.

Fear of Diagnosis or Treatment: Concerns about potential diagnoses or complicated treatments can deter men from seeking medical attention, leading to delayed diagnosis and worsening conditions.

Strategies for Empowering Men to Prioritize Sexual Health

1. Open Communication and Education: Encourage open and honest conversations about sexual health among men, both individually and within their relationships. Normalize discussions about sexual concerns, preferences, and challenges to foster a supportive environment.

2. Promote Regular Checkups: Encourage men to schedule regular checkups with their healthcare providers, including pelvic exams and screening for sexually transmitted infections (STIs). Early detection and intervention can prevent complications and improve overall health.

3. Address Underlying Issues: Recognize that sexual health concerns can stem from underlying physical or psychological factors, such as stress, anxiety, or depression. Address these underlying issues to improve overall well-being and sexual function.

4. Embrace Healthy Lifestyle: Encourage men to adopt healthy lifestyle habits, including regular exercise, a balanced diet, and adequate sleep. These habits can improve physical and mental health, positively impacting sexual function.

5. Seek Professional Support: Encourage men to seek professional help when needed, whether from a healthcare provider, therapist, or sexual health specialist. They can provide personalized guidance, address specific concerns, and offer treatment options.

6. Normalize Sexual Health Conversations: Integrate sexual health discussions into routine healthcare visits and public health campaigns. Make sexual health information easily accessible and encourage men to ask questions without judgment.

7. Promote Body Positivity: Encourage men to embrace body positivity and self-acceptance, regardless of societal beauty standards. Positive body image can boost self-esteem and confidence, enhancing sexual well-being.

8. Address Cultural Influences: Recognize the impact of cultural and religious beliefs on men's sexual health.

Provide culturally sensitive and inclusive information and support to address specific needs and concerns.

Empowering men to take charge of their sexual health is an ongoing process that requires open communication, education, and support. By breaking down barriers, promoting awareness, and providing accessible resources, we can create a culture where men feel empowered to prioritize their sexual health and maintain fulfilling and healthy relationships.

www.ingramcontent.com/pod-product-compliance
Lightning Source LLC
Chambersburg PA
CBHW070943260726
48661CB00003B/1102